I've learned through running and racing over the years that self-confidence is a major key to success. I hope this book helps guide you to become a more confident person and runner!

xo Steph

GOAL SETTING

WHAT WOULD YOU LIKE TO ACHIEVE THIS YEAR?

WHAT WOULD YOU LIKE TO ACHIEVE IN THE NEXT 5 YEARS?

WHAT STEPS ARE YOU GOING TO TAKE TO ACHIEVE THESE GOALS?

PERSONAL RECORDS

5K:

8K:

10K:

HALF MARATHON:

MARATHON:

UPCOMING RACES:

"Racing is the fun part,
it's the reward for all
of the hard work."

-Kara Goucher

WEEK OF:

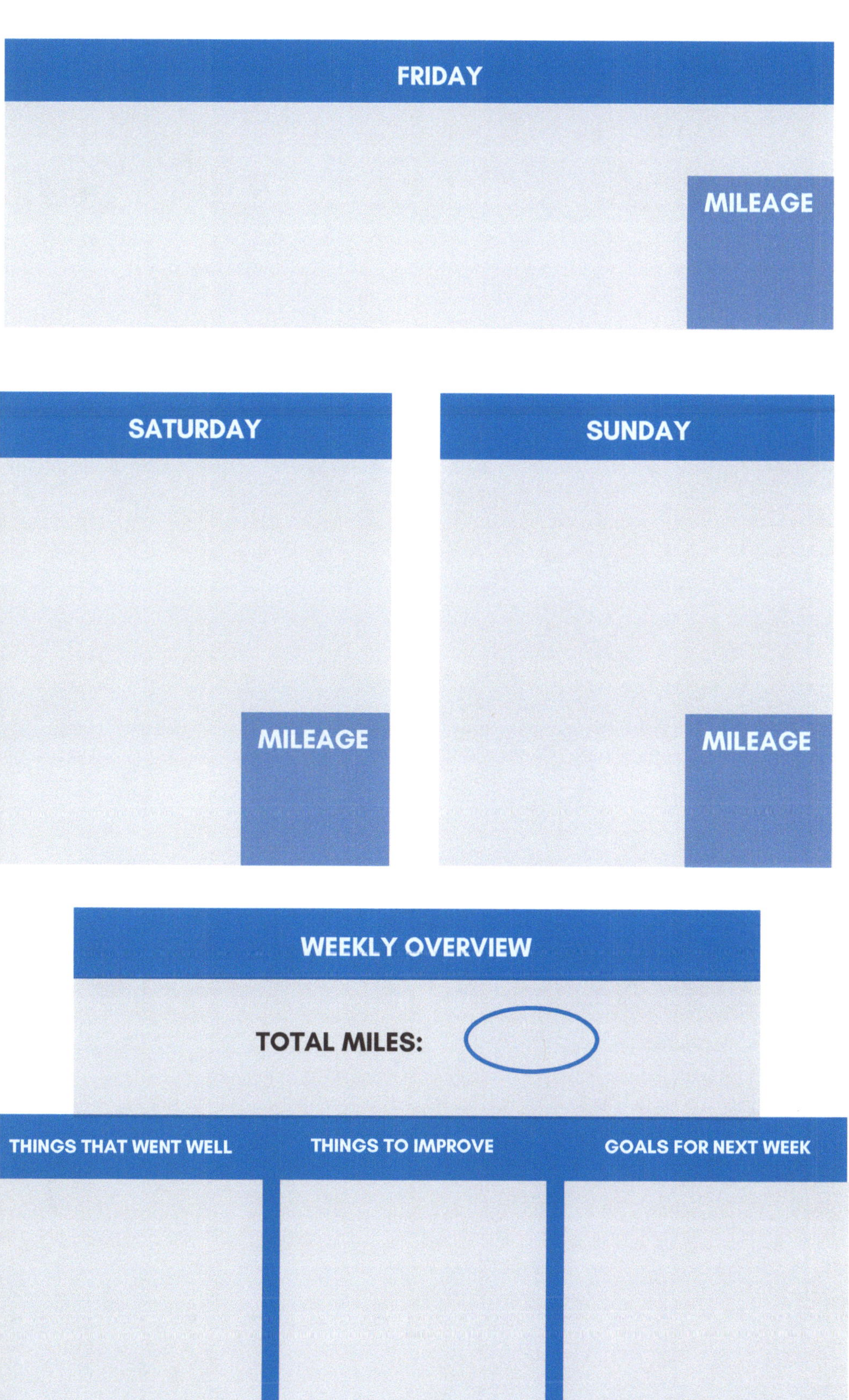
FRIDAY
MILEAGE
SATURDAY
MILEAGE
SUNDAY
MILEAGE
WEEKLY OVERVIEW
TOTAL MILES:
THINGS THAT WENT WELL
THINGS TO IMPROVE
GOALS FOR NEXT WEEK

WEEK OF:

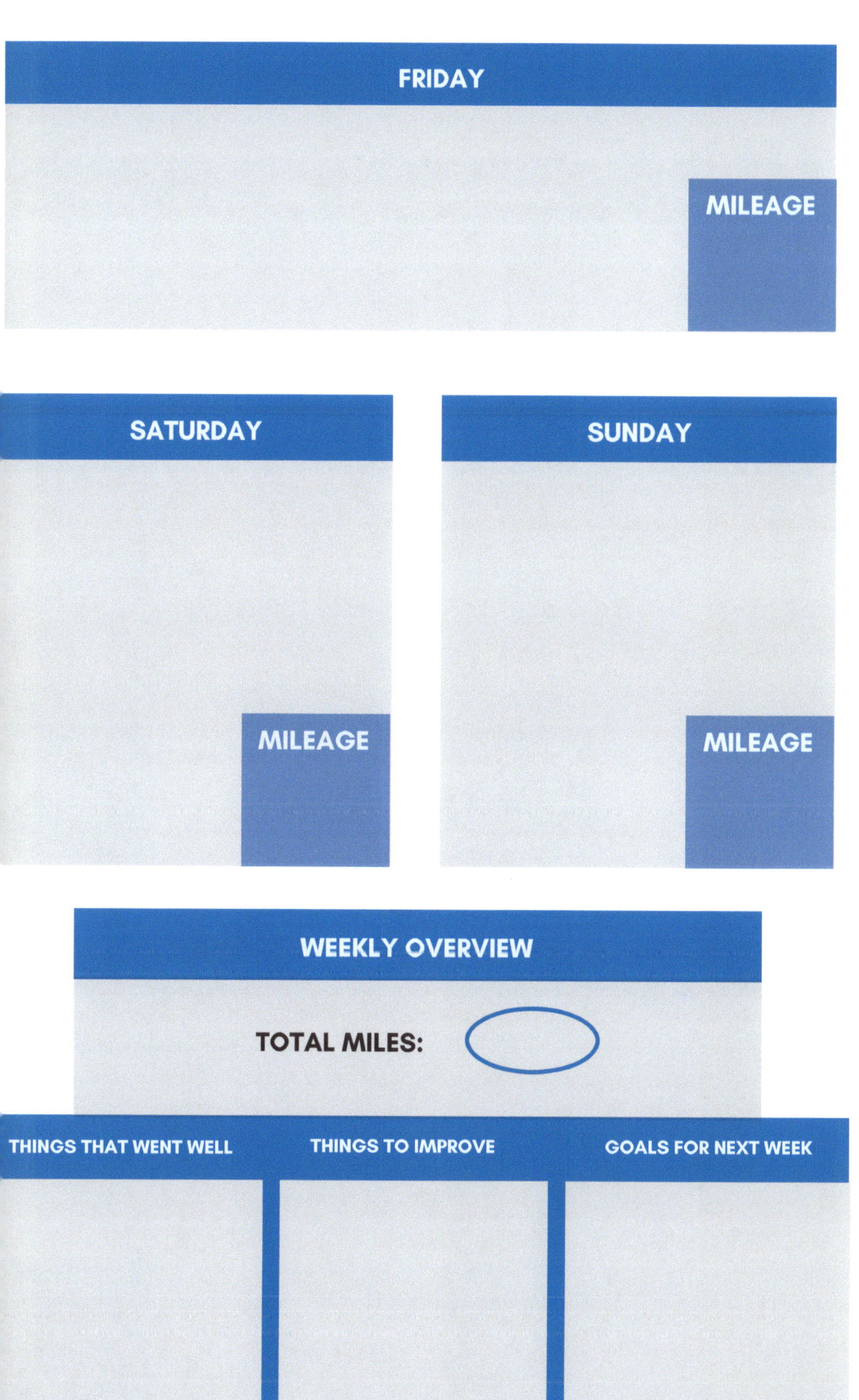

FRIDAY
MILEAGE
SATURDAY
MILEAGE
SUNDAY
MILEAGE
WEEKLY OVERVIEW
TOTAL MILES:
THINGS THAT WENT WELL
THINGS TO IMPROVE
GOALS FOR NEXT WEEK

WEEK OF:

MANTRA OF THE WEEK

MONDAY

MILEAGE

TUESDAY

MILEAGE

WEDNESDAY

MILEAGE

THURSDAY

MILEAGE

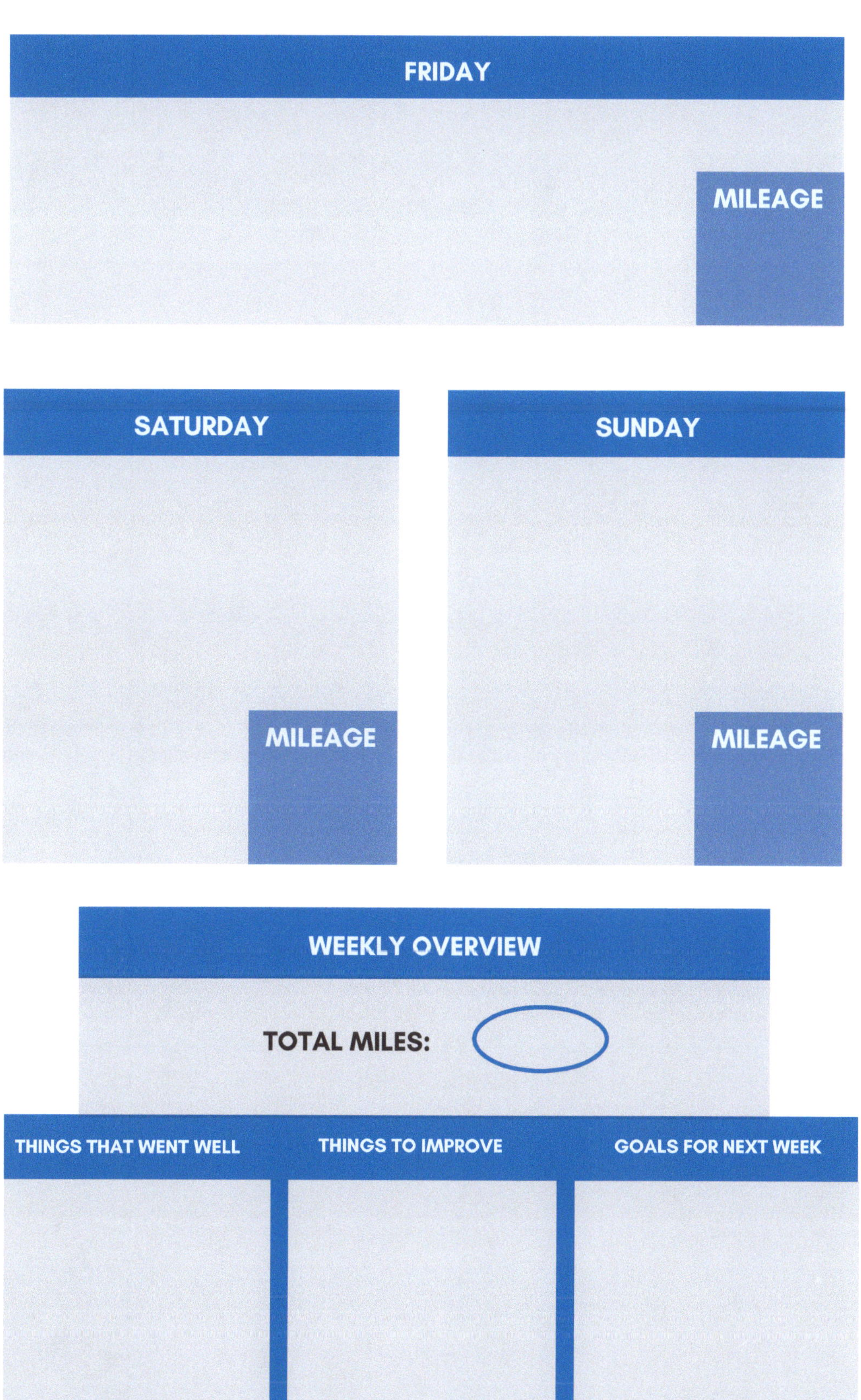

FRIDAY
MILEAGE
SATURDAY
MILEAGE
SUNDAY
MILEAGE
WEEKLY OVERVIEW
TOTAL MILES:
THINGS THAT WENT WELL
THINGS TO IMPROVE
GOALS FOR NEXT WEEK

WEEK OF:

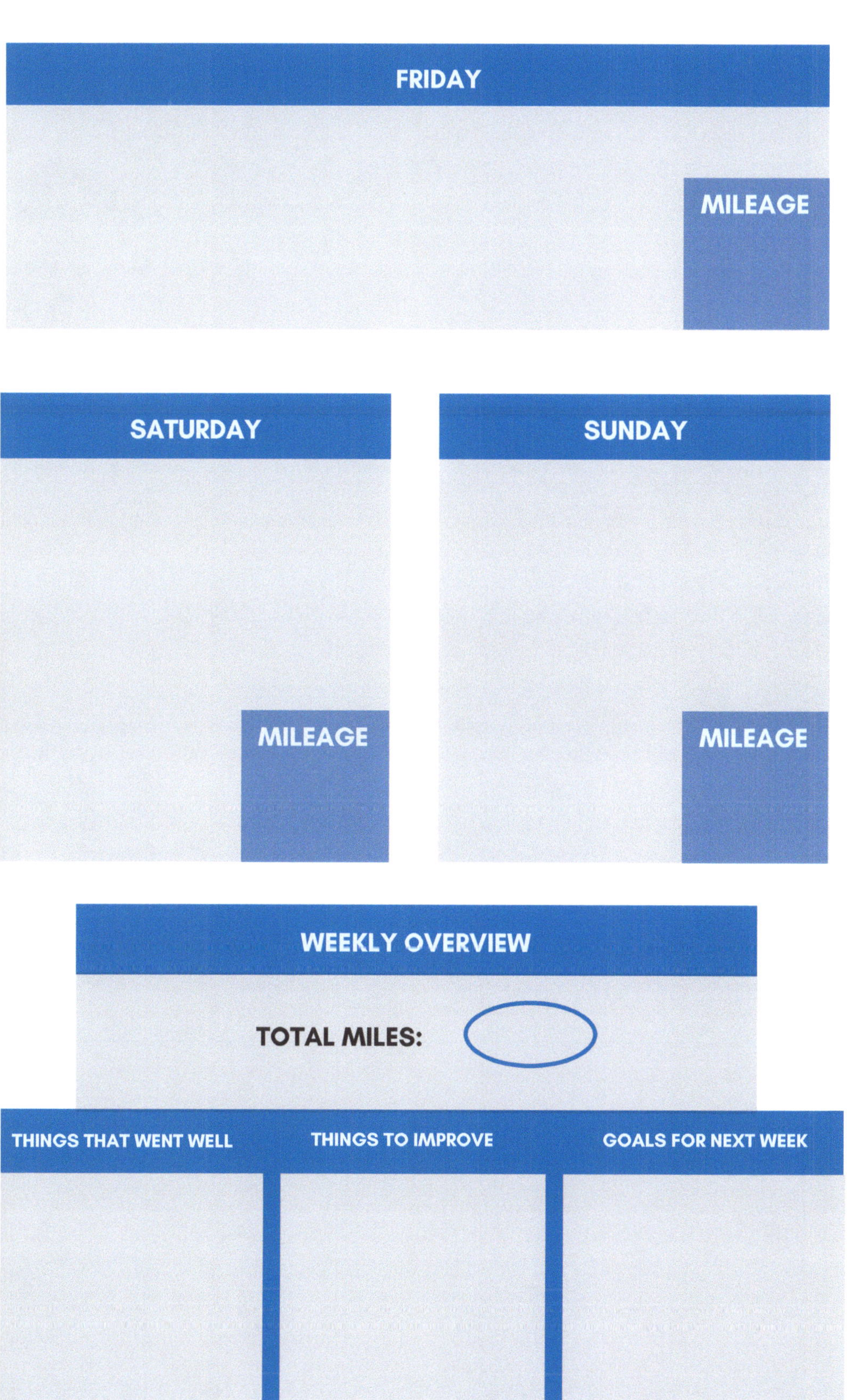
FRIDAY
MILEAGE
SATURDAY
MILEAGE
SUNDAY
MILEAGE
WEEKLY OVERVIEW
TOTAL MILES:
THINGS THAT WENT WELL
THINGS TO IMPROVE
GOALS FOR NEXT WEEK

WEEK OF:

MANTRA OF THE WEEK

MONDAY

MILEAGE

TUESDAY

MILEAGE

WEDNESDAY

MILEAGE

THURSDAY

MILEAGE

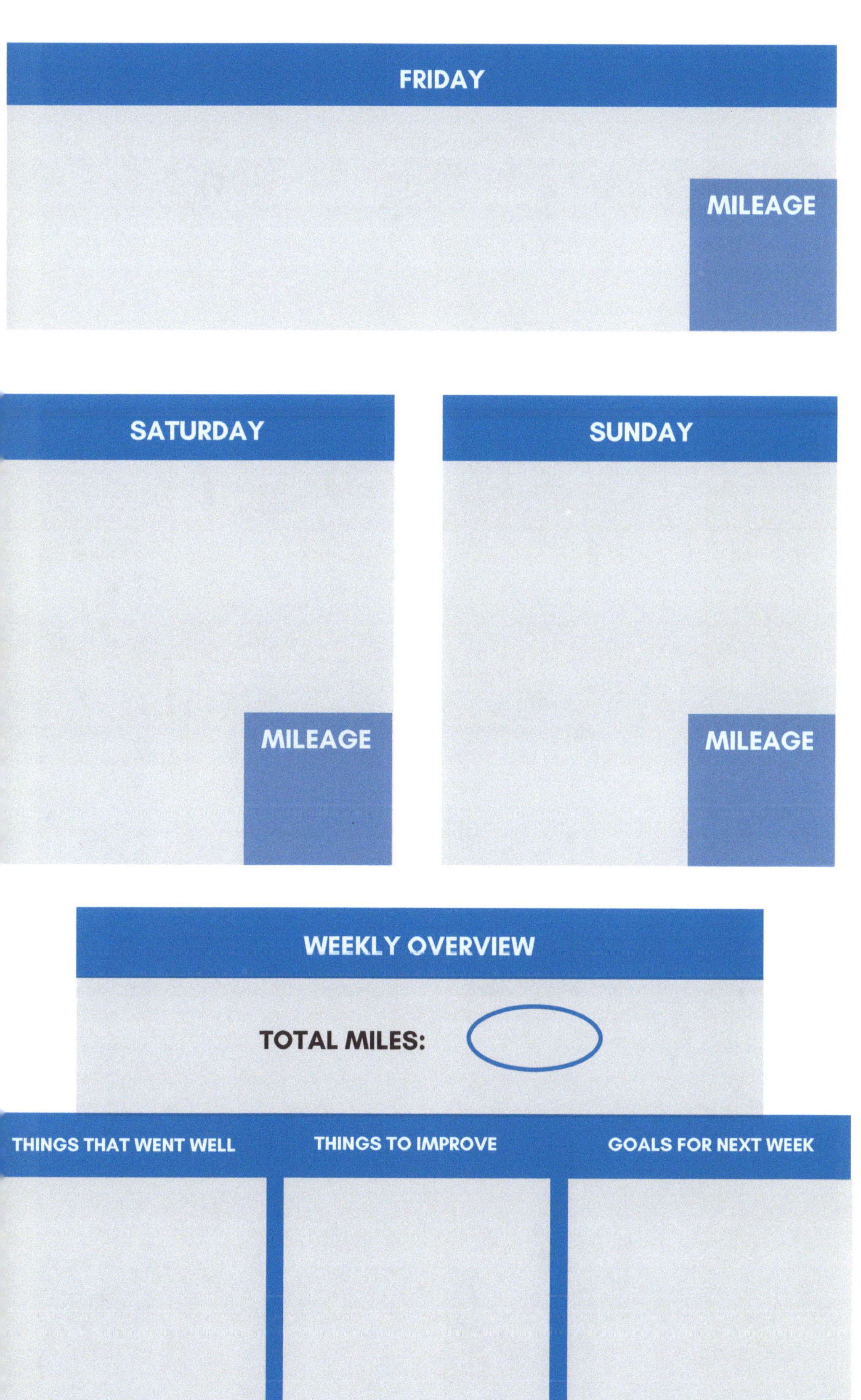

FRIDAY
MILEAGE
SATURDAY
MILEAGE
SUNDAY
MILEAGE
WEEKLY OVERVIEW
TOTAL MILES:
THINGS THAT WENT WELL
THINGS TO IMPROVE
GOALS FOR NEXT WEEK

WEEK OF:

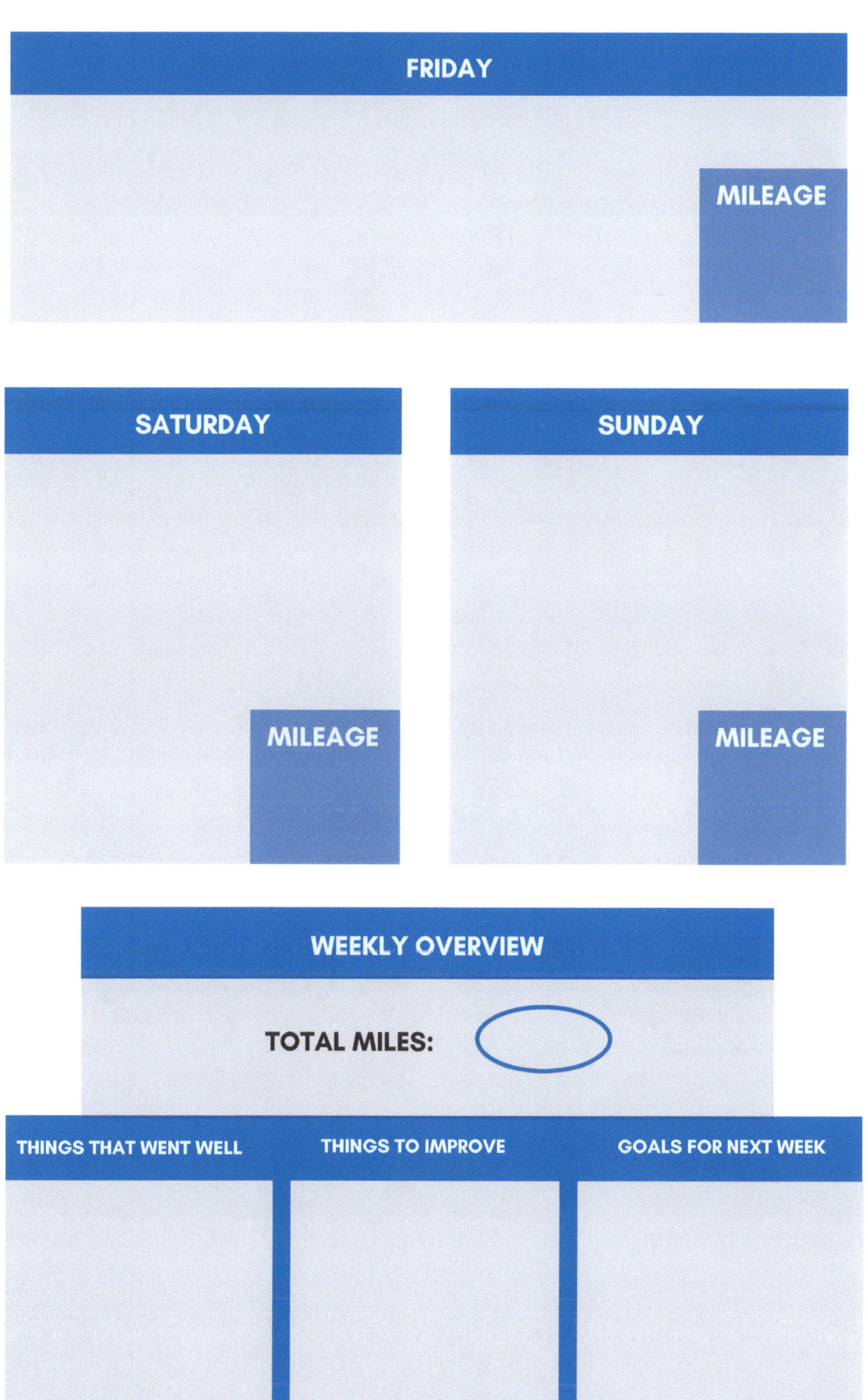

FRIDAY
MILEAGE
SATURDAY
MILEAGE
SUNDAY
MILEAGE
WEEKLY OVERVIEW
TOTAL MILES:
THINGS THAT WENT WELL
THINGS TO IMPROVE
GOALS FOR NEXT WEEK

WEEK OF:

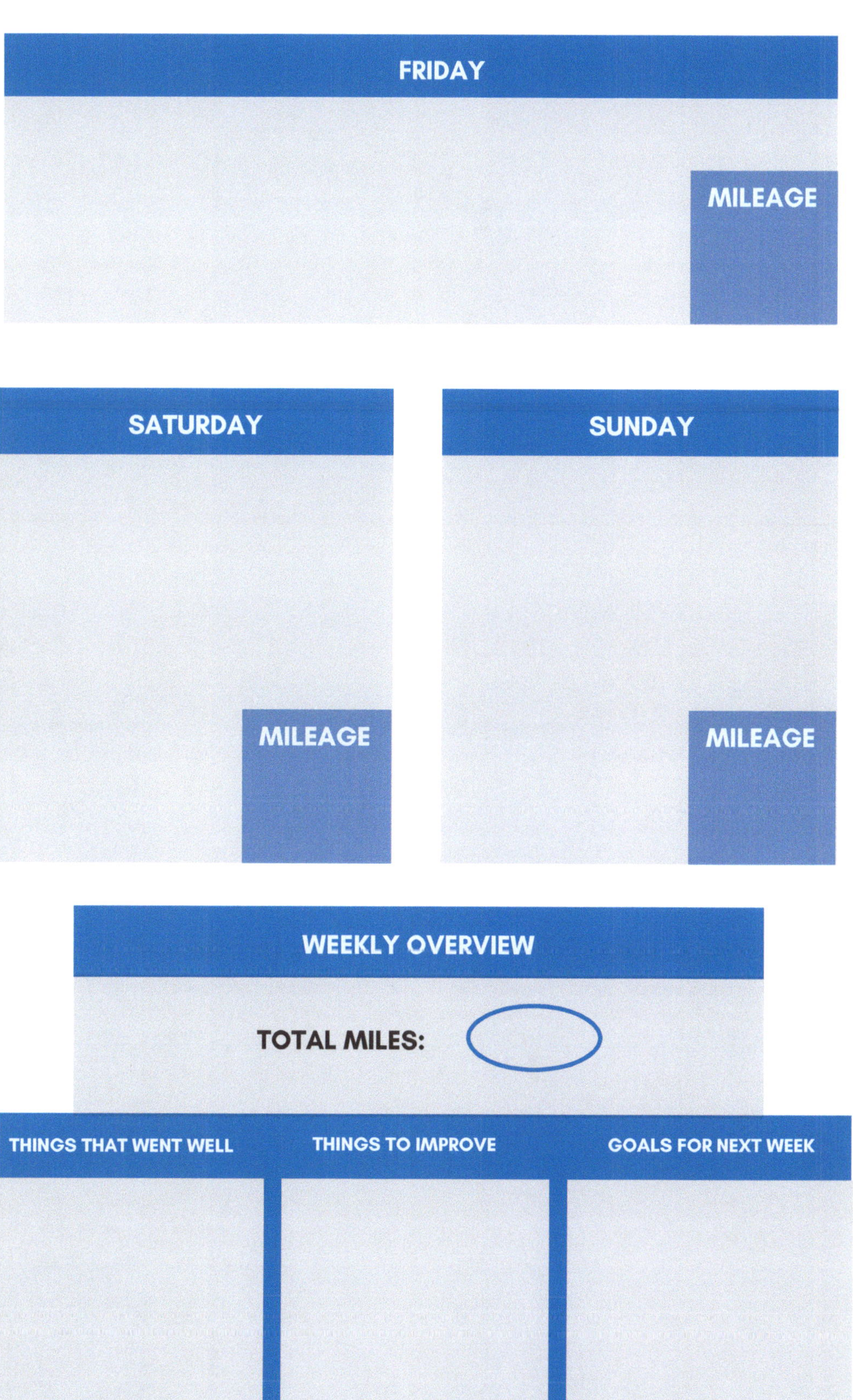

FRIDAY
MILEAGE
SATURDAY
MILEAGE
SUNDAY
MILEAGE
WEEKLY OVERVIEW
TOTAL MILES:
THINGS THAT WENT WELL
THINGS TO IMPROVE
GOALS FOR NEXT WEEK

WEEK OF:

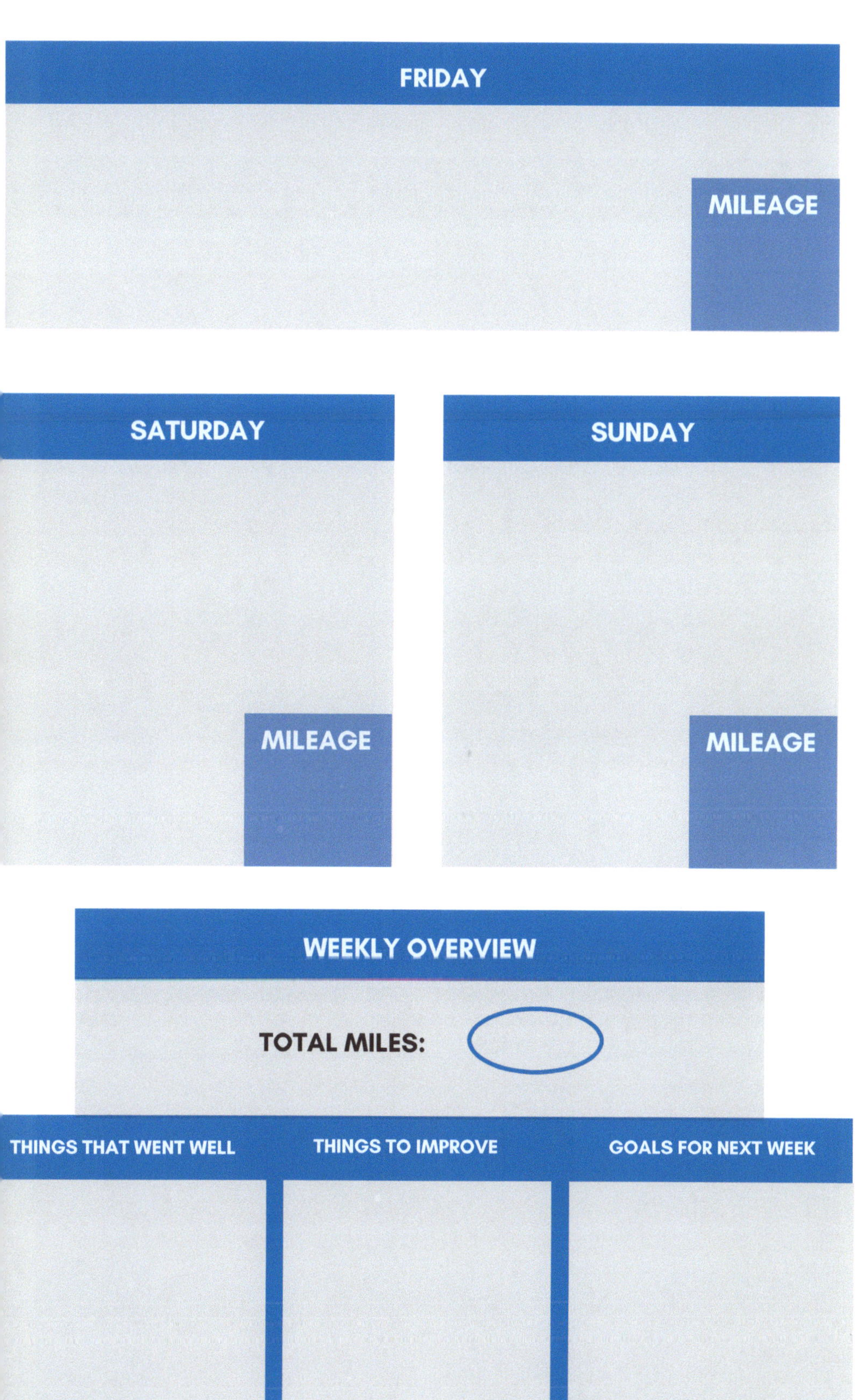

FRIDAY
MILEAGE
SATURDAY
MILEAGE
SUNDAY
MILEAGE
WEEKLY OVERVIEW
TOTAL MILES:
THINGS THAT WENT WELL
THINGS TO IMPROVE
GOALS FOR NEXT WEEK

WEEK OF:

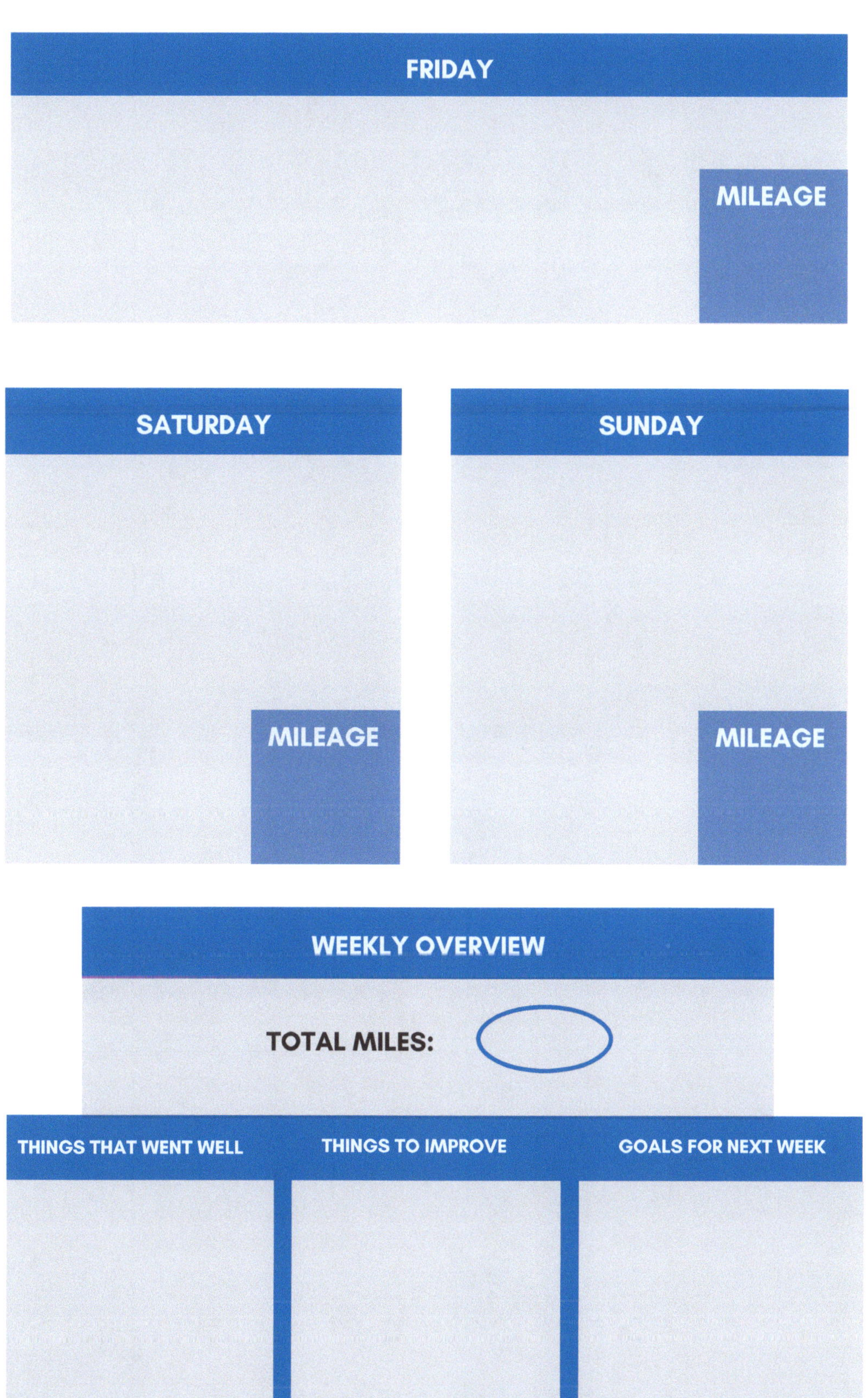

FRIDAY
MILEAGE
SATURDAY
MILEAGE
SUNDAY
MILEAGE
WEEKLY OVERVIEW
TOTAL MILES:
THINGS THAT WENT WELL
THINGS TO IMPROVE
GOALS FOR NEXT WEEK

WEEK OF:

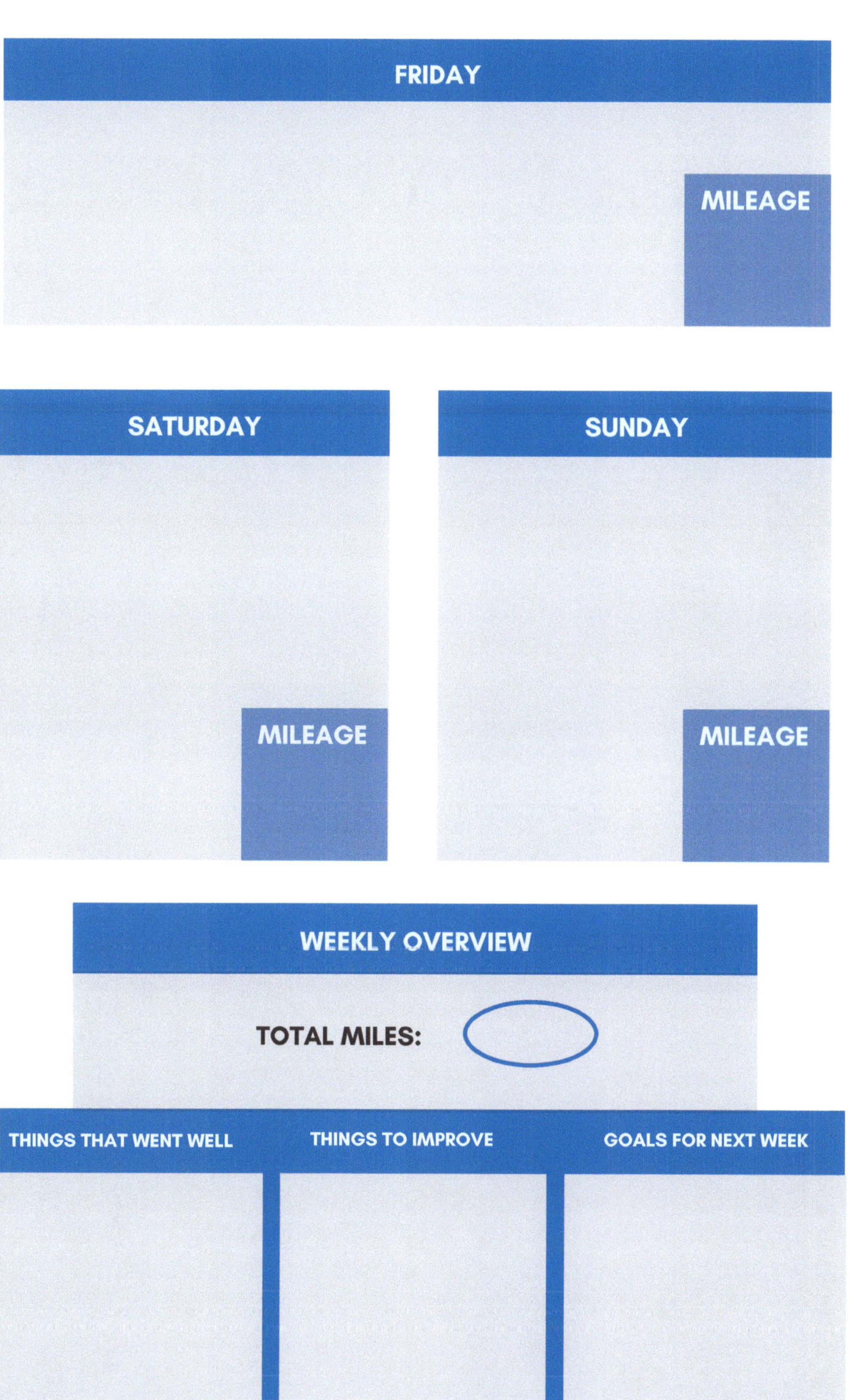

FRIDAY
MILEAGE
SATURDAY
MILEAGE
SUNDAY
MILEAGE
WEEKLY OVERVIEW
TOTAL MILES:
THINGS THAT WENT WELL
THINGS TO IMPROVE
GOALS FOR NEXT WEEK

WEEK OF:

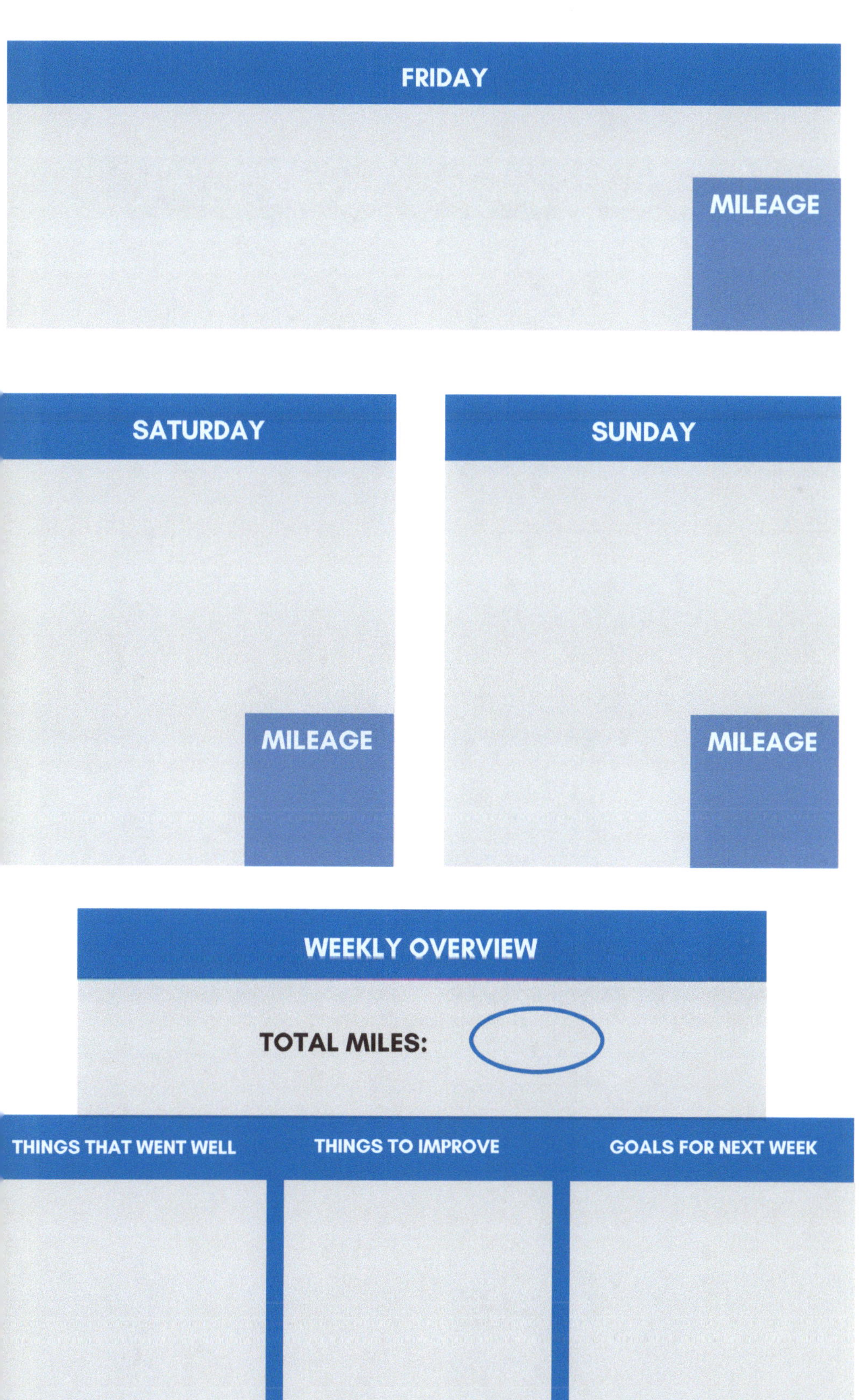
FRIDAY
MILEAGE
SATURDAY
MILEAGE
SUNDAY
MILEAGE
WEEKLY OVERVIEW
TOTAL MILES:
THINGS THAT WENT WELL
THINGS TO IMPROVE
GOALS FOR NEXT WEEK

WEEK OF:

MANTRA OF THE WEEK

MONDAY

TUESDAY

MILEAGE

MILEAGE

WEDNESDAY

THURSDAY

MILEAGE

MILEAGE

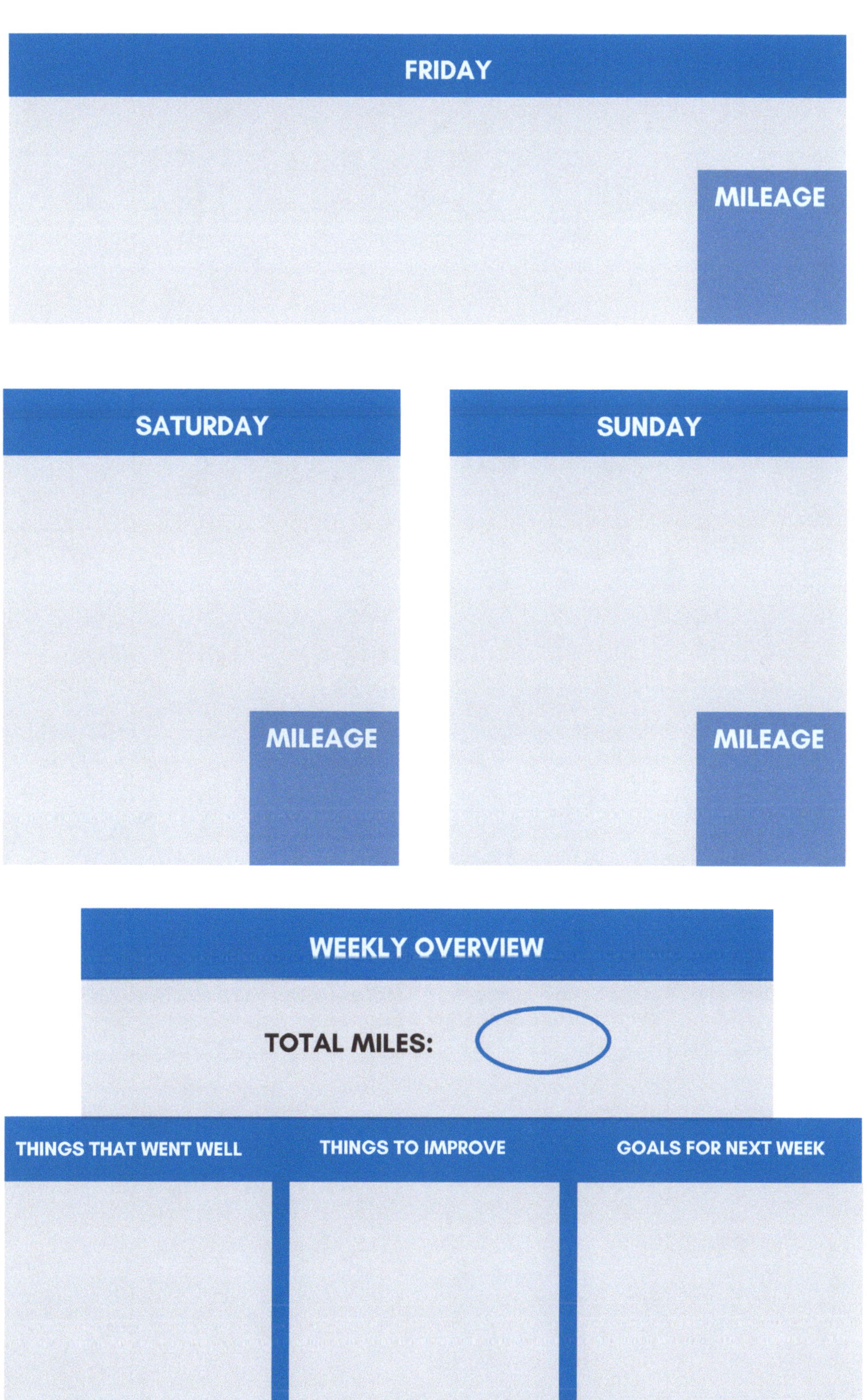

FRIDAY
MILEAGE
SATURDAY
MILEAGE
SUNDAY
MILEAGE
WEEKLY OVERVIEW
TOTAL MILES:
THINGS THAT WENT WELL
THINGS TO IMPROVE
GOALS FOR NEXT WEEK

WEEK OF:

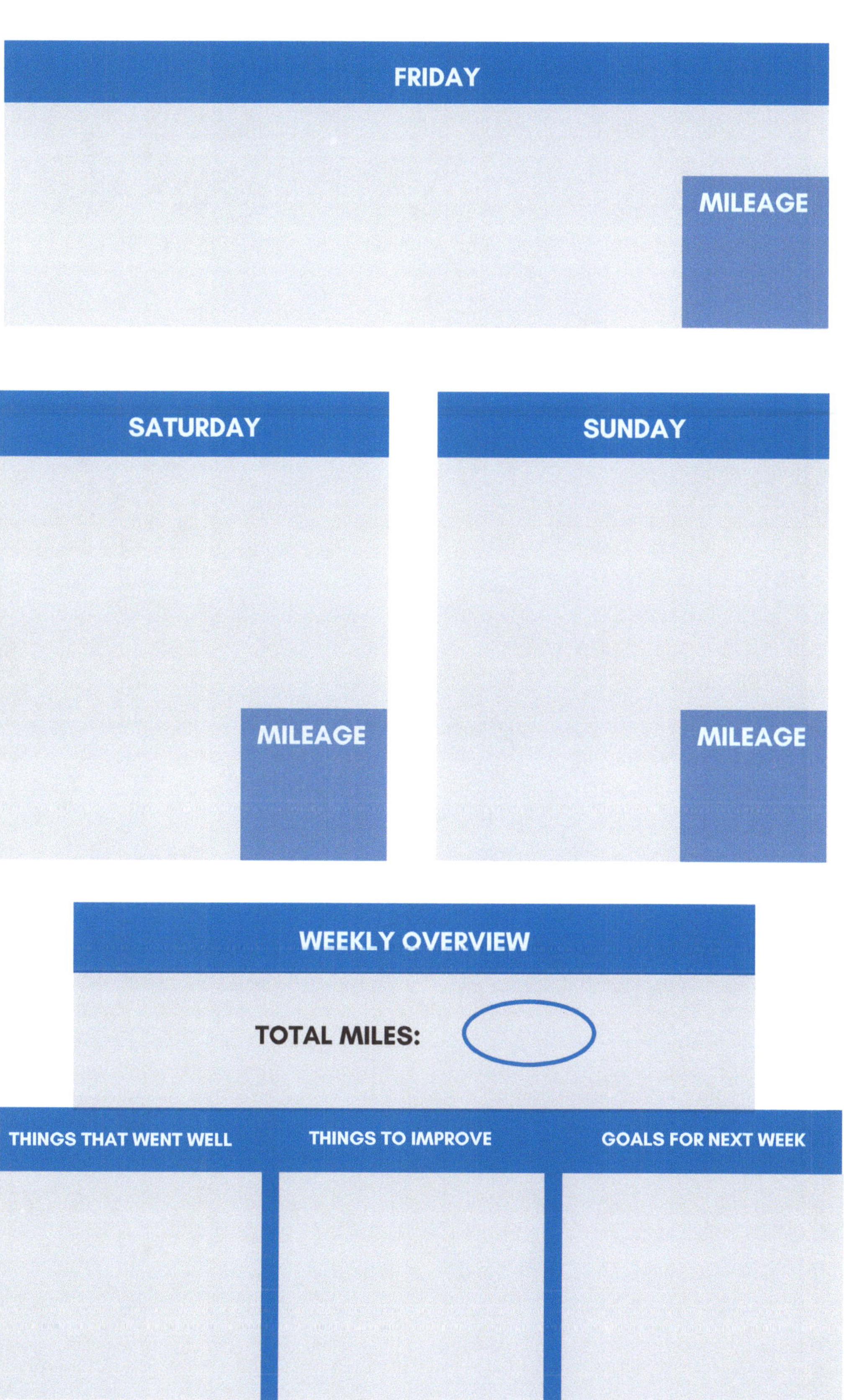
FRIDAY
MILEAGE
SATURDAY
MILEAGE
SUNDAY
MILEAGE
WEEKLY OVERVIEW
TOTAL MILES:
THINGS THAT WENT WELL
THINGS TO IMPROVE
GOALS FOR NEXT WEEK

WEEK OF:

MANTRA OF THE WEEK

MONDAY

MILEAGE

TUESDAY

MILEAGE

WEDNESDAY

MILEAGE

THURSDAY

MILEAGE

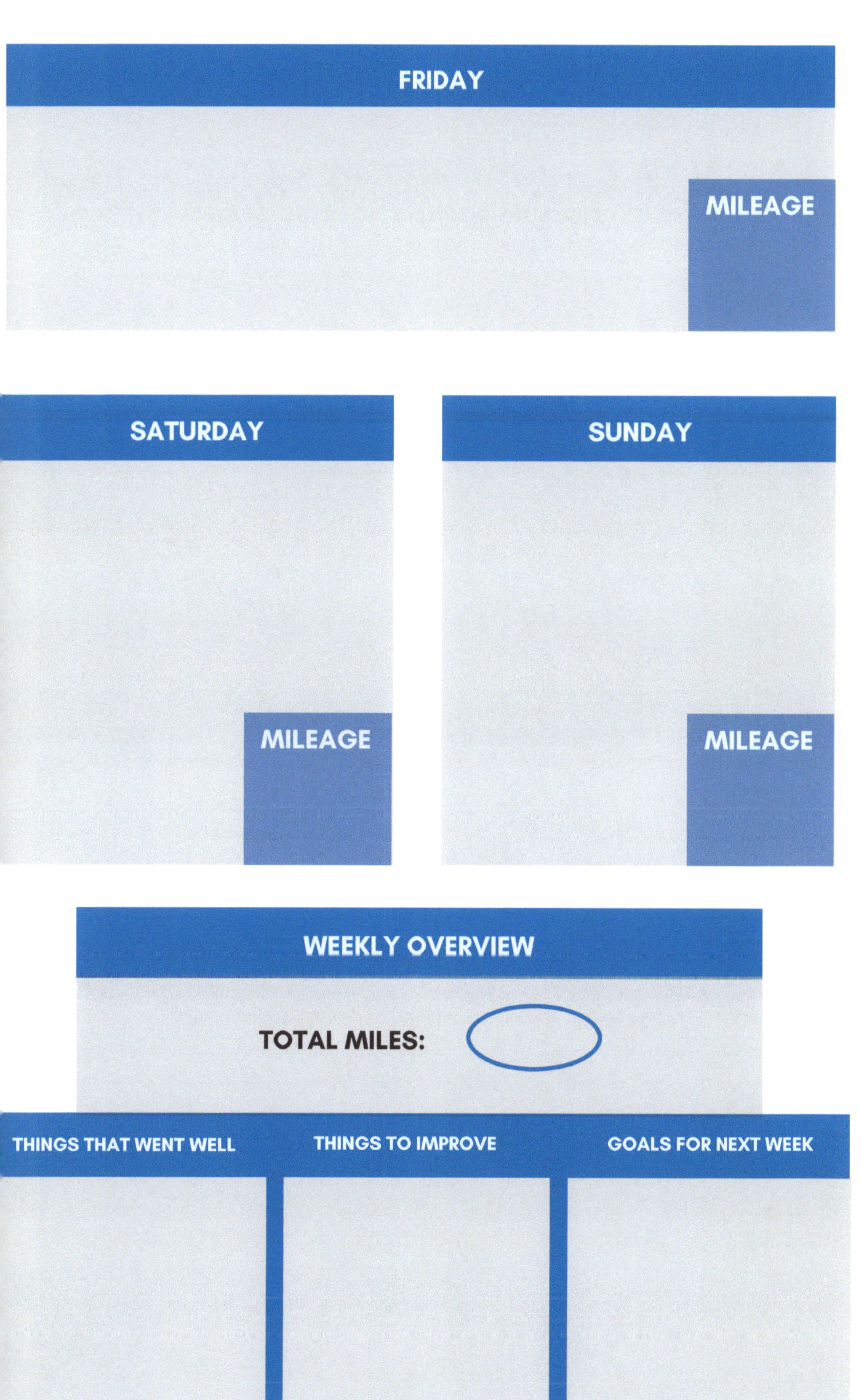

FRIDAY
MILEAGE
SATURDAY
MILEAGE
SUNDAY
MILEAGE
WEEKLY OVERVIEW
TOTAL MILES:
THINGS THAT WENT WELL
THINGS TO IMPROVE
GOALS FOR NEXT WEEK

WEEK OF:

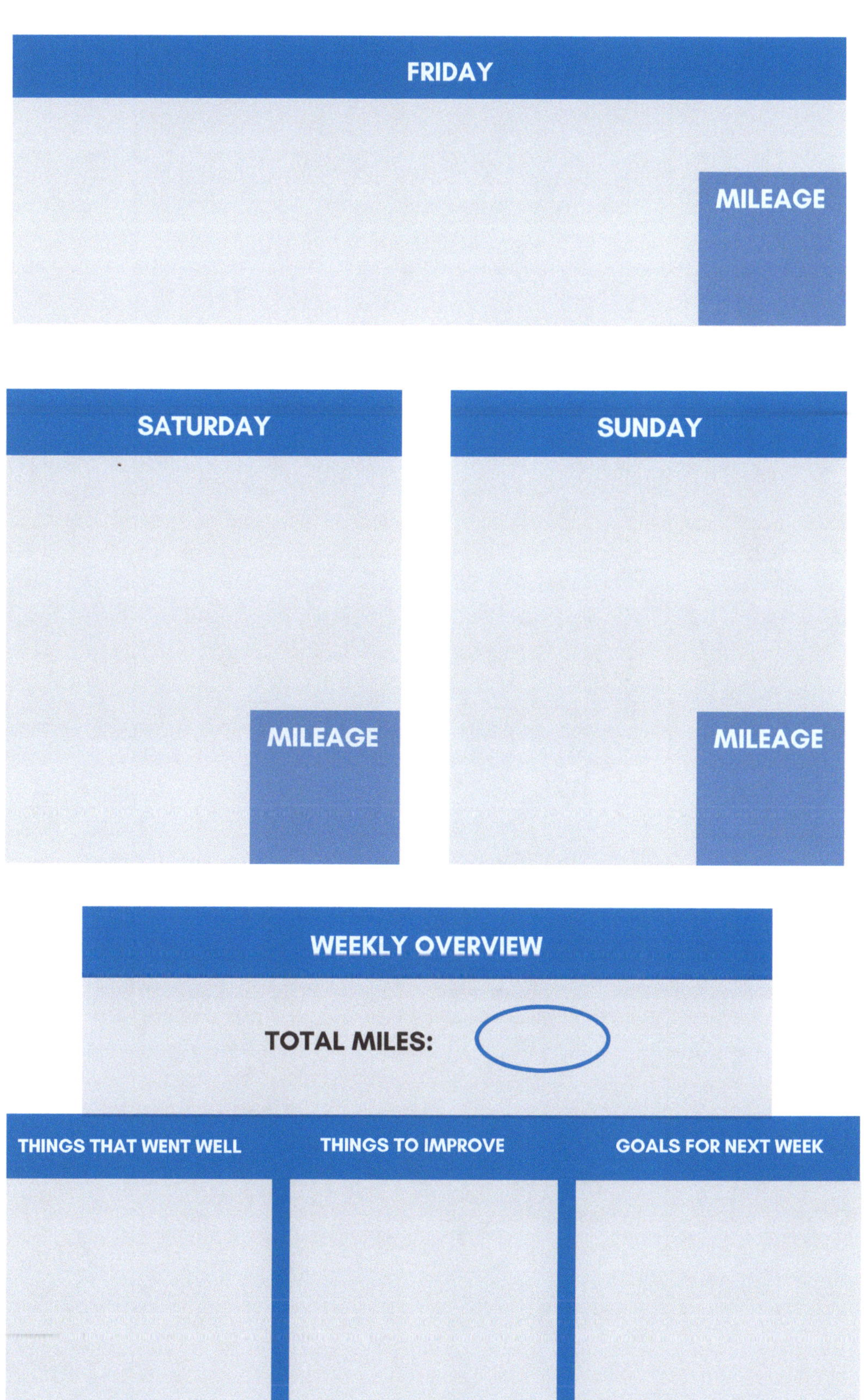
FRIDAY
MILEAGE
SATURDAY
MILEAGE
SUNDAY
MILEAGE
WEEKLY OVERVIEW
TOTAL MILES:
THINGS THAT WENT WELL
THINGS TO IMPROVE
GOALS FOR NEXT WEEK

WEEK OF:

MANTRA OF THE WEEK

MONDAY

MILEAGE

TUESDAY

MILEAGE

WEDNESDAY

MILEAGE

THURSDAY

MILEAGE

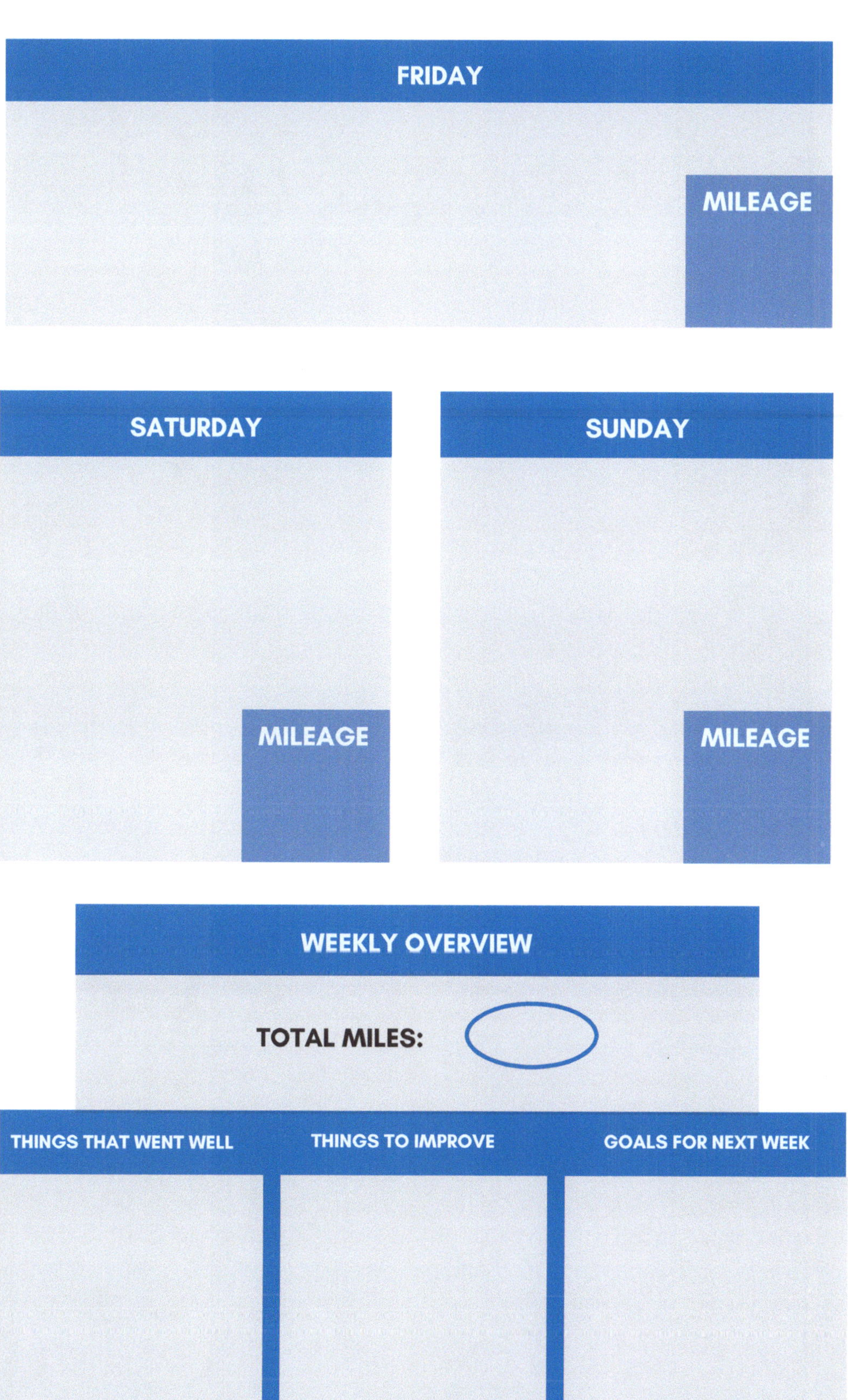
FRIDAY
MILEAGE
SATURDAY
MILEAGE
SUNDAY
MILEAGE
WEEKLY OVERVIEW
TOTAL MILES:
THINGS THAT WENT WELL
THINGS TO IMPROVE
GOALS FOR NEXT WEEK

WEEK OF:

MANTRA OF THE WEEK

MONDAY

TUESDAY

MILEAGE

MILEAGE

WEDNESDAY

THURSDAY

MILEAGE

MILEAGE

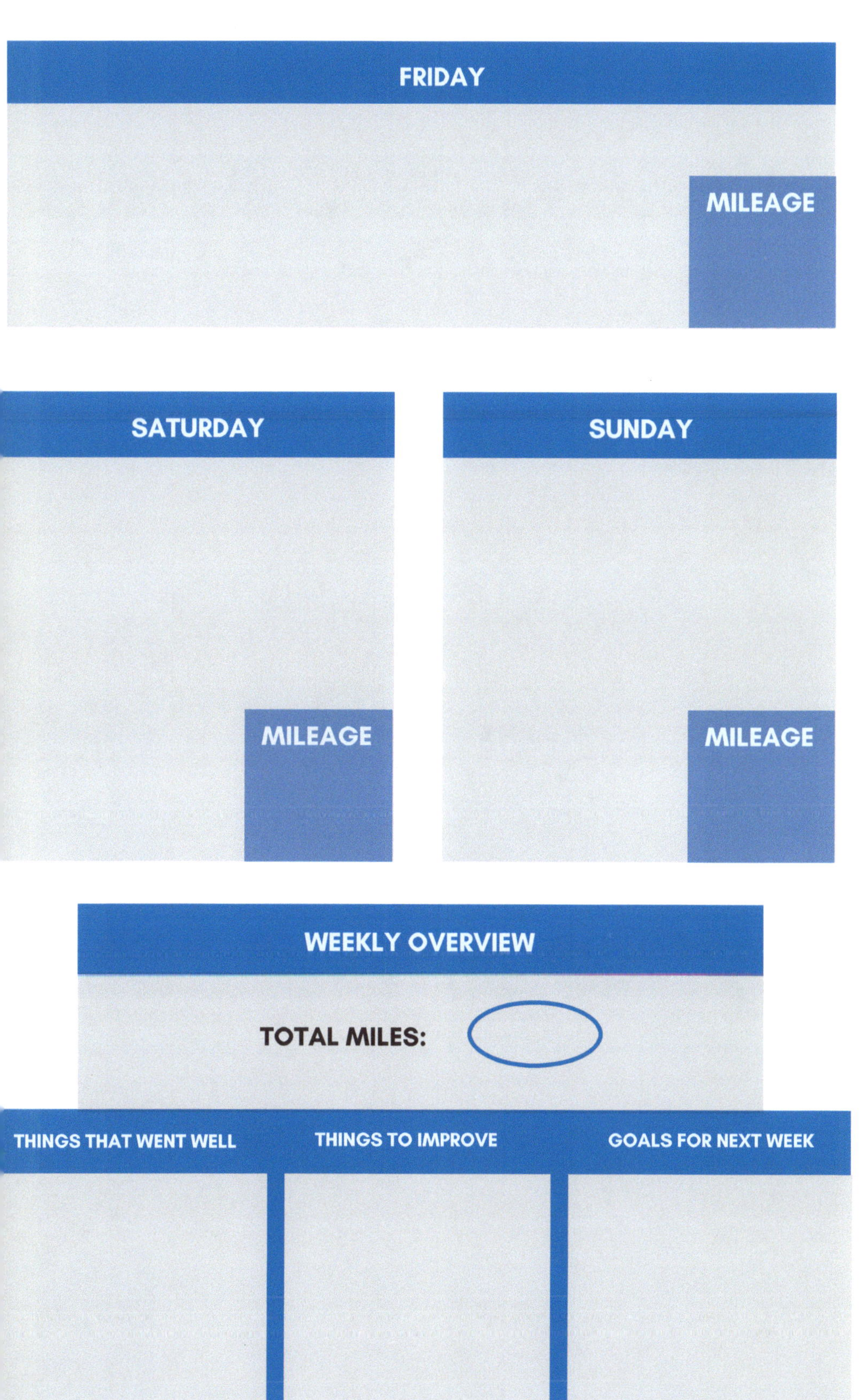

FRIDAY
MILEAGE
SATURDAY
MILEAGE
SUNDAY
MILEAGE
WEEKLY OVERVIEW
TOTAL MILES:
THINGS THAT WENT WELL
THINGS TO IMPROVE
GOALS FOR NEXT WEEK

WEEK OF:

MANTRA OF THE WEEK

MONDAY

TUESDAY

MILEAGE

MILEAGE

WEDNESDAY

THURSDAY

MILEAGE

MILEAGE

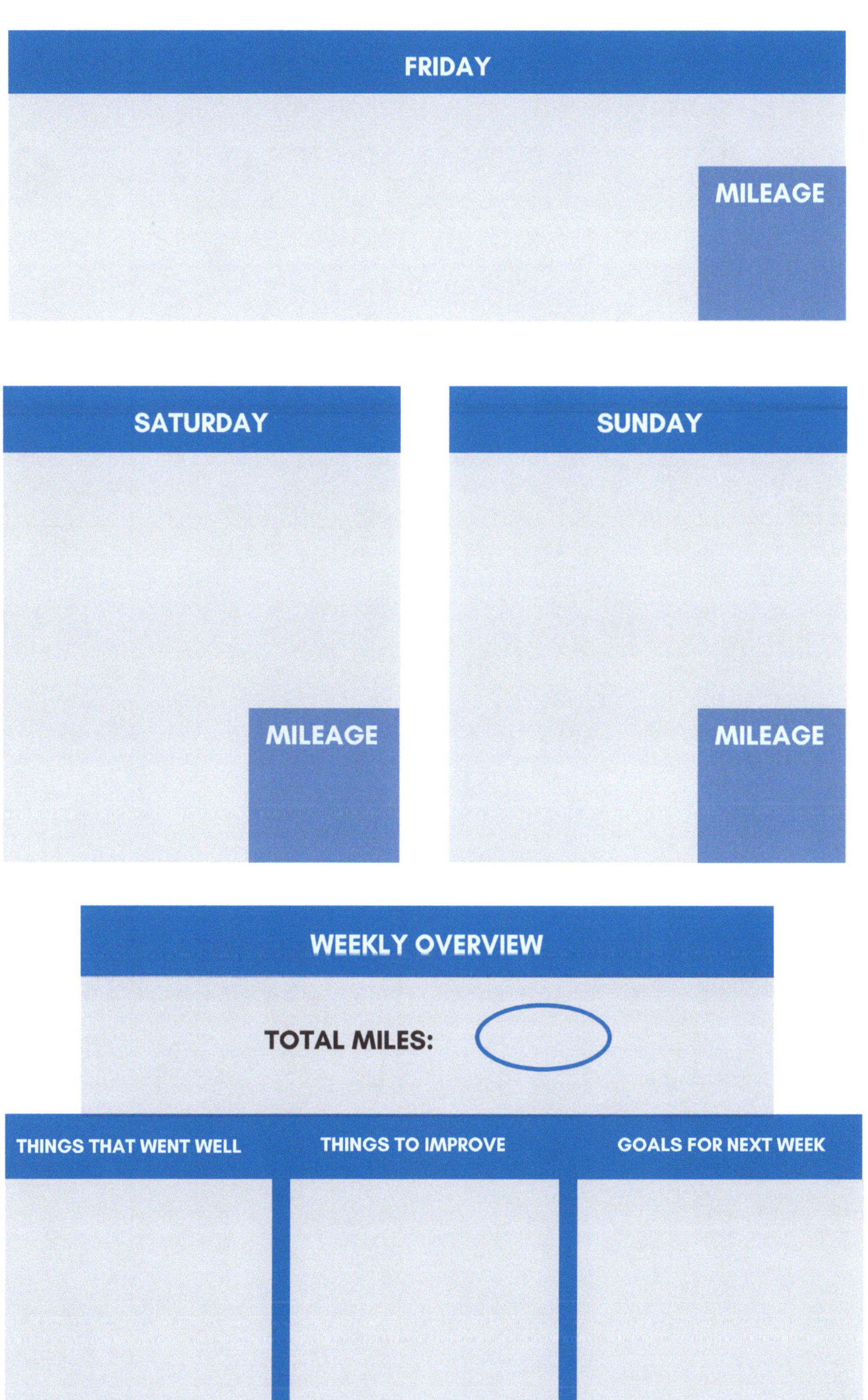

FRIDAY
MILEAGE
SATURDAY
MILEAGE
SUNDAY
MILEAGE
WEEKLY OVERVIEW
TOTAL MILES:
THINGS THAT WENT WELL
THINGS TO IMPROVE
GOALS FOR NEXT WEEK

WEEK OF:

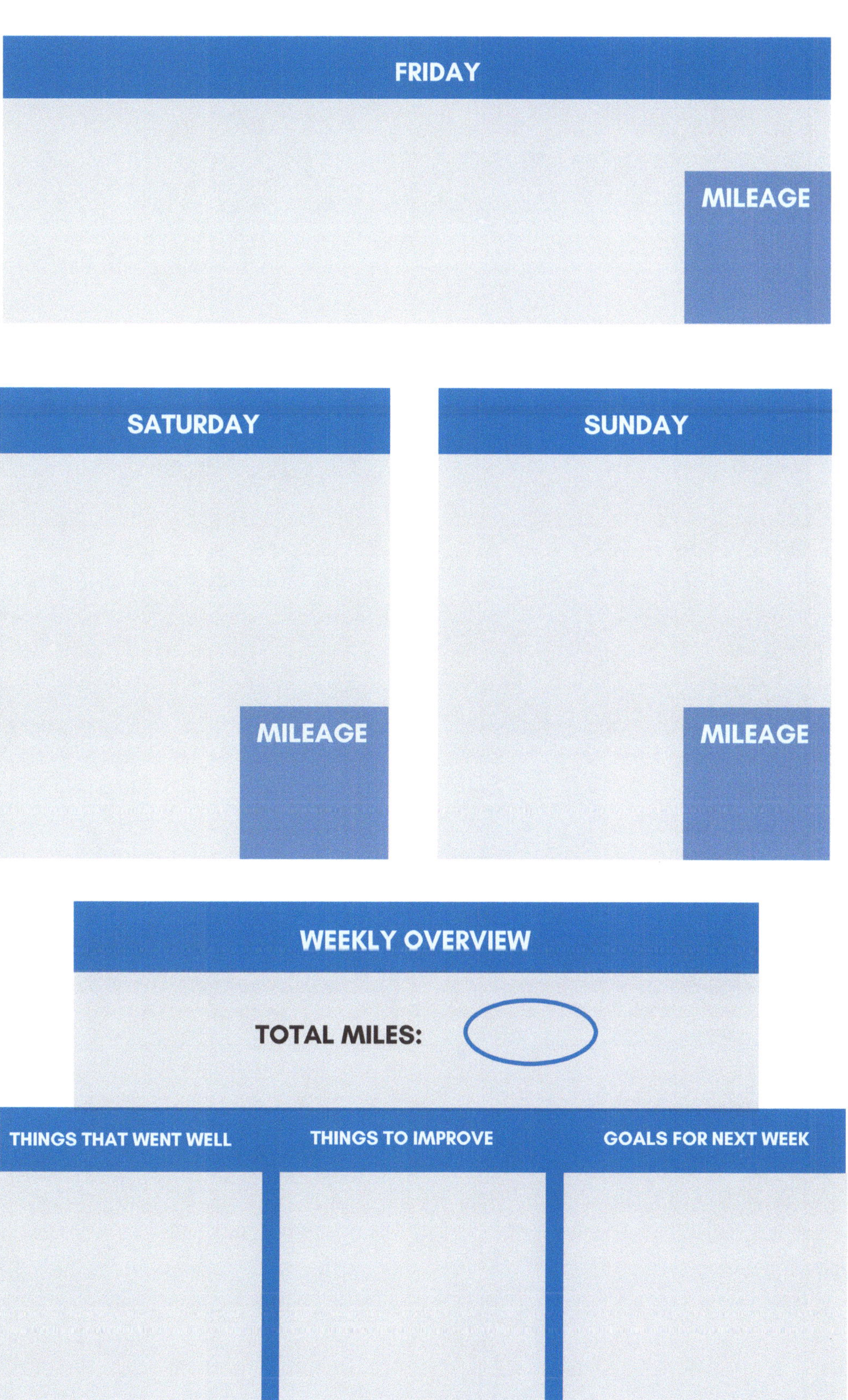

FRIDAY
MILEAGE
SATURDAY
MILEAGE
SUNDAY
MILEAGE
WEEKLY OVERVIEW
TOTAL MILES:
THINGS THAT WENT WELL
THINGS TO IMPROVE
GOALS FOR NEXT WEEK

WEEK OF:

MANTRA OF THE WEEK

MONDAY

MILEAGE

TUESDAY

MILEAGE

WEDNESDAY

MILEAGE

THURSDAY

MILEAGE

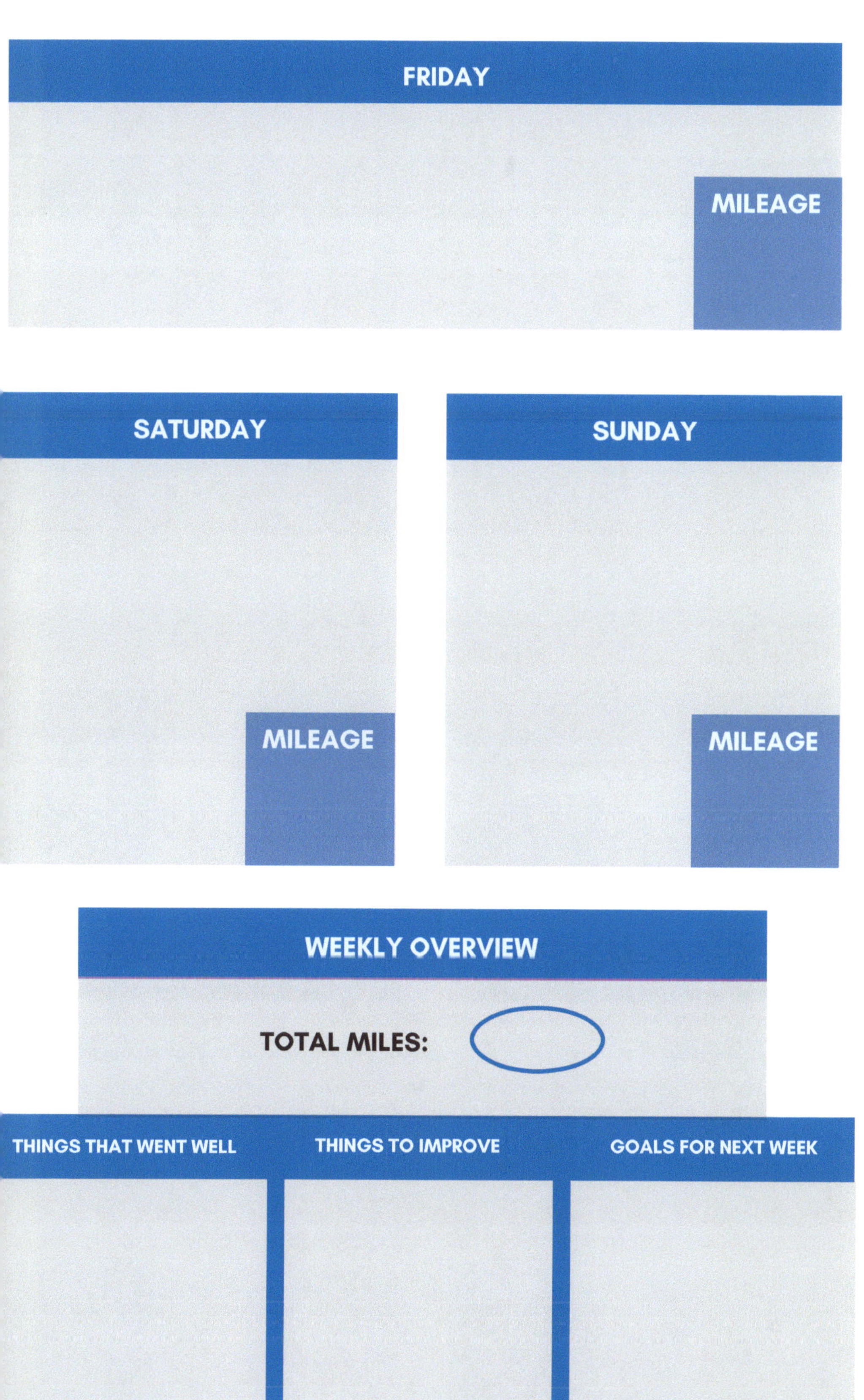

FRIDAY
MILEAGE
SATURDAY
MILEAGE
SUNDAY
MILEAGE
WEEKLY OVERVIEW
TOTAL MILES:
THINGS THAT WENT WELL
THINGS TO IMPROVE
GOALS FOR NEXT WEEK

WEEK OF:

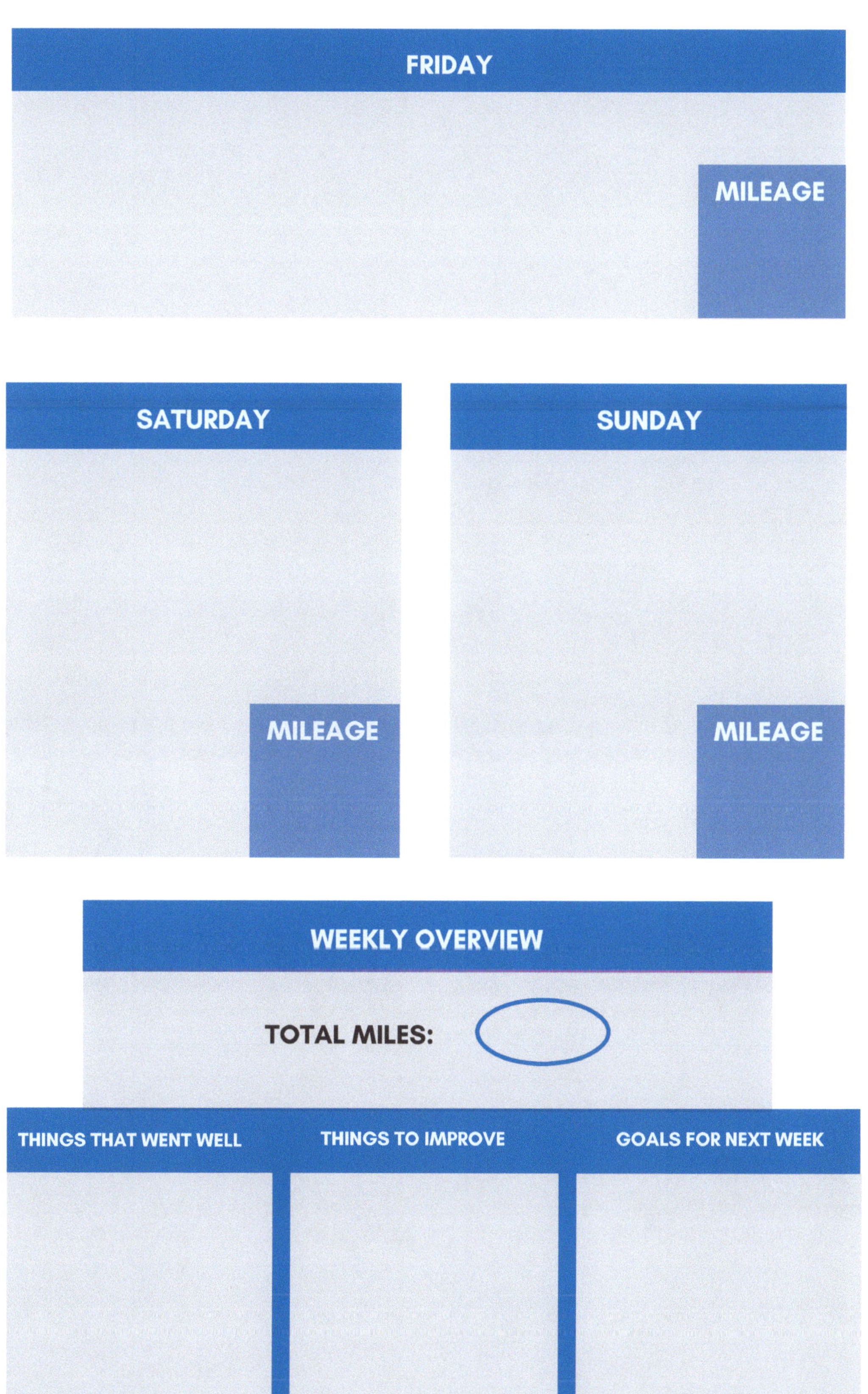

FRIDAY
MILEAGE
SATURDAY
MILEAGE
SUNDAY
MILEAGE
WEEKLY OVERVIEW
TOTAL MILES:
THINGS THAT WENT WELL
THINGS TO IMPROVE
GOALS FOR NEXT WEEK

WEEK OF:

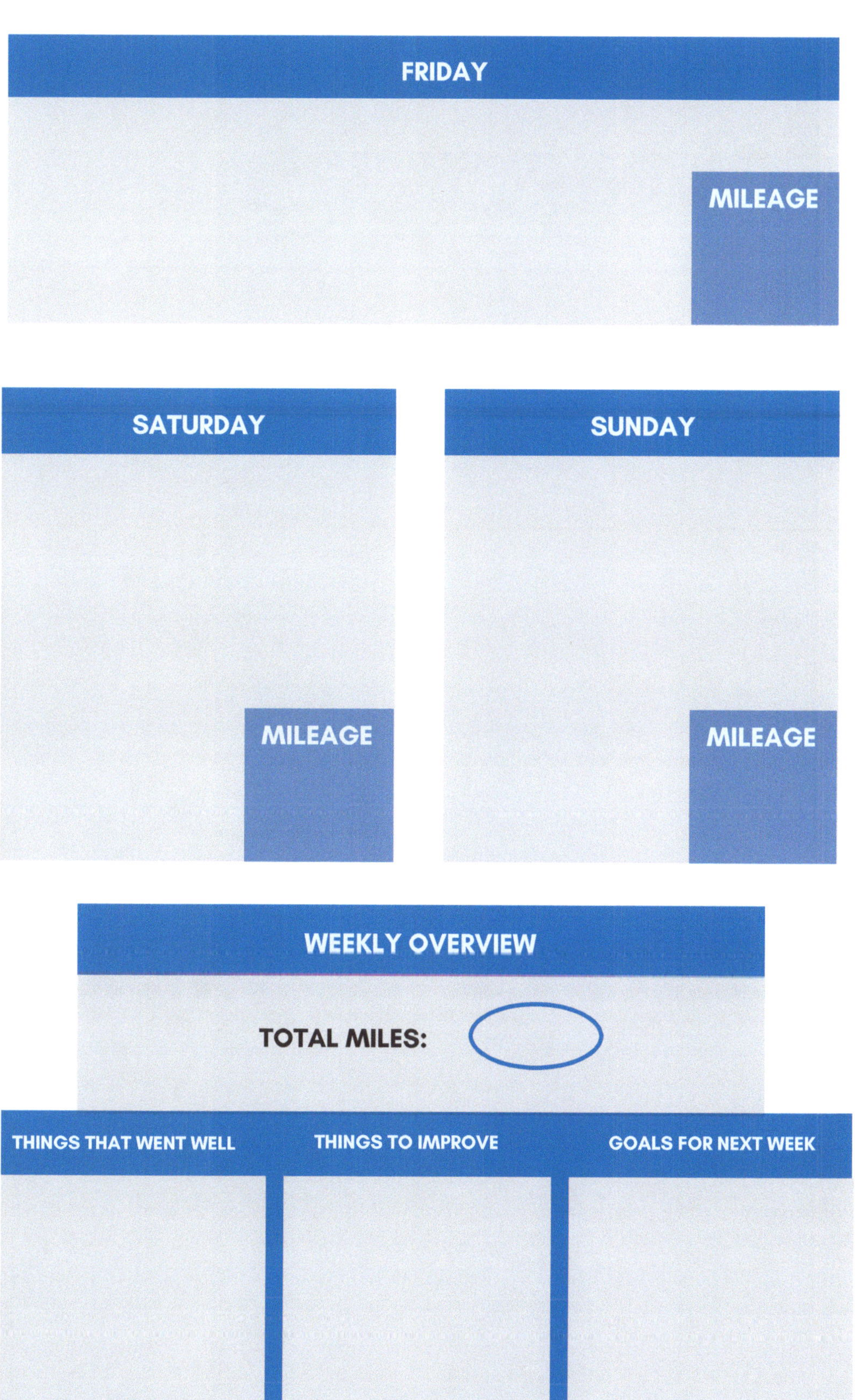

FRIDAY
MILEAGE
SATURDAY
MILEAGE
SUNDAY
MILEAGE
WEEKLY OVERVIEW
TOTAL MILES:
THINGS THAT WENT WELL
THINGS TO IMPROVE
GOALS FOR NEXT WEEK

WEEK OF:

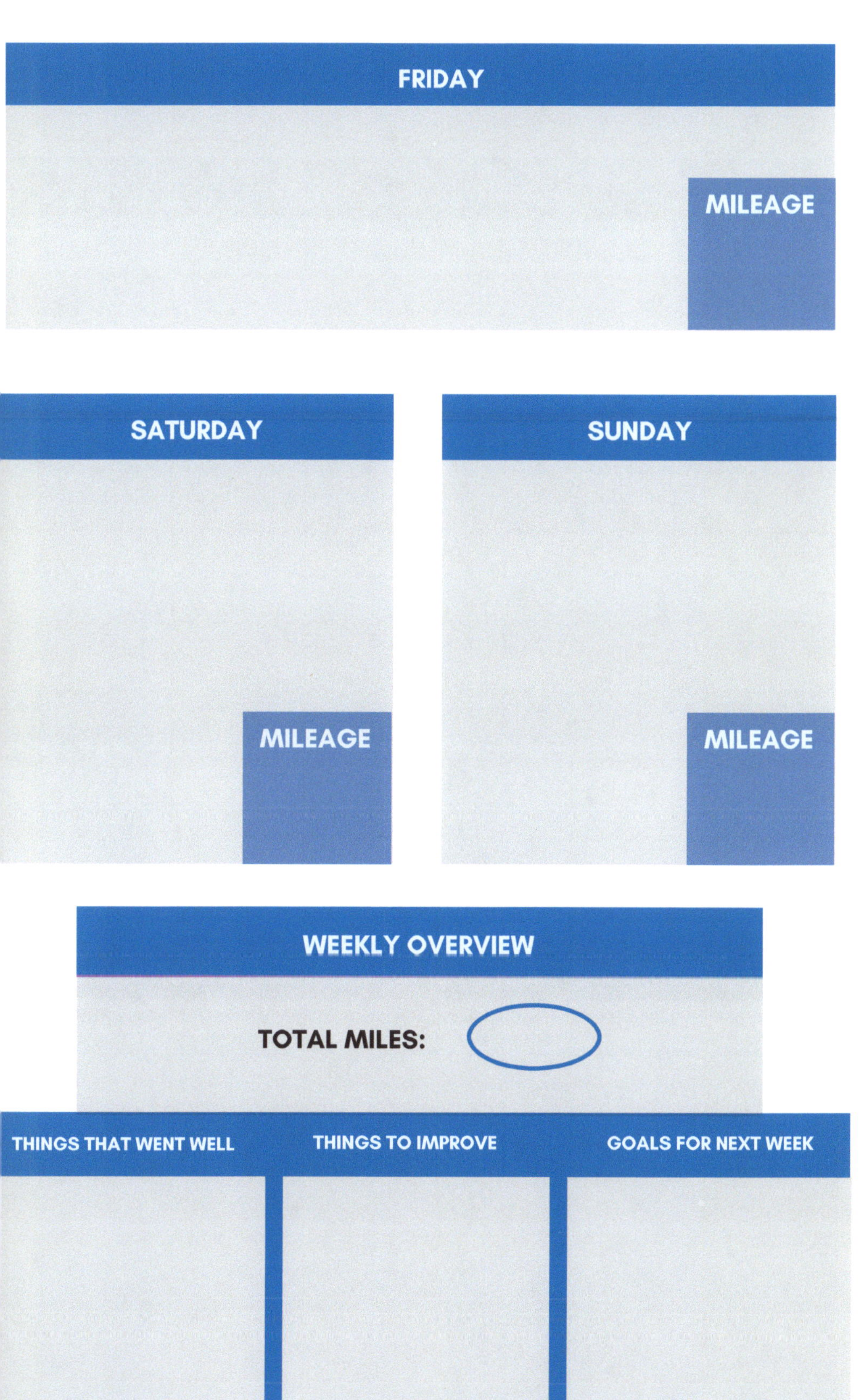

FRIDAY
MILEAGE
SATURDAY
MILEAGE
SUNDAY
MILEAGE
WEEKLY OVERVIEW
TOTAL MILES:
THINGS THAT WENT WELL
THINGS TO IMPROVE
GOALS FOR NEXT WEEK

WEEK OF:

MANTRA OF THE WEEK

MONDAY

MILEAGE

TUESDAY

MILEAGE

WEDNESDAY

MILEAGE

THURSDAY

MILEAGE

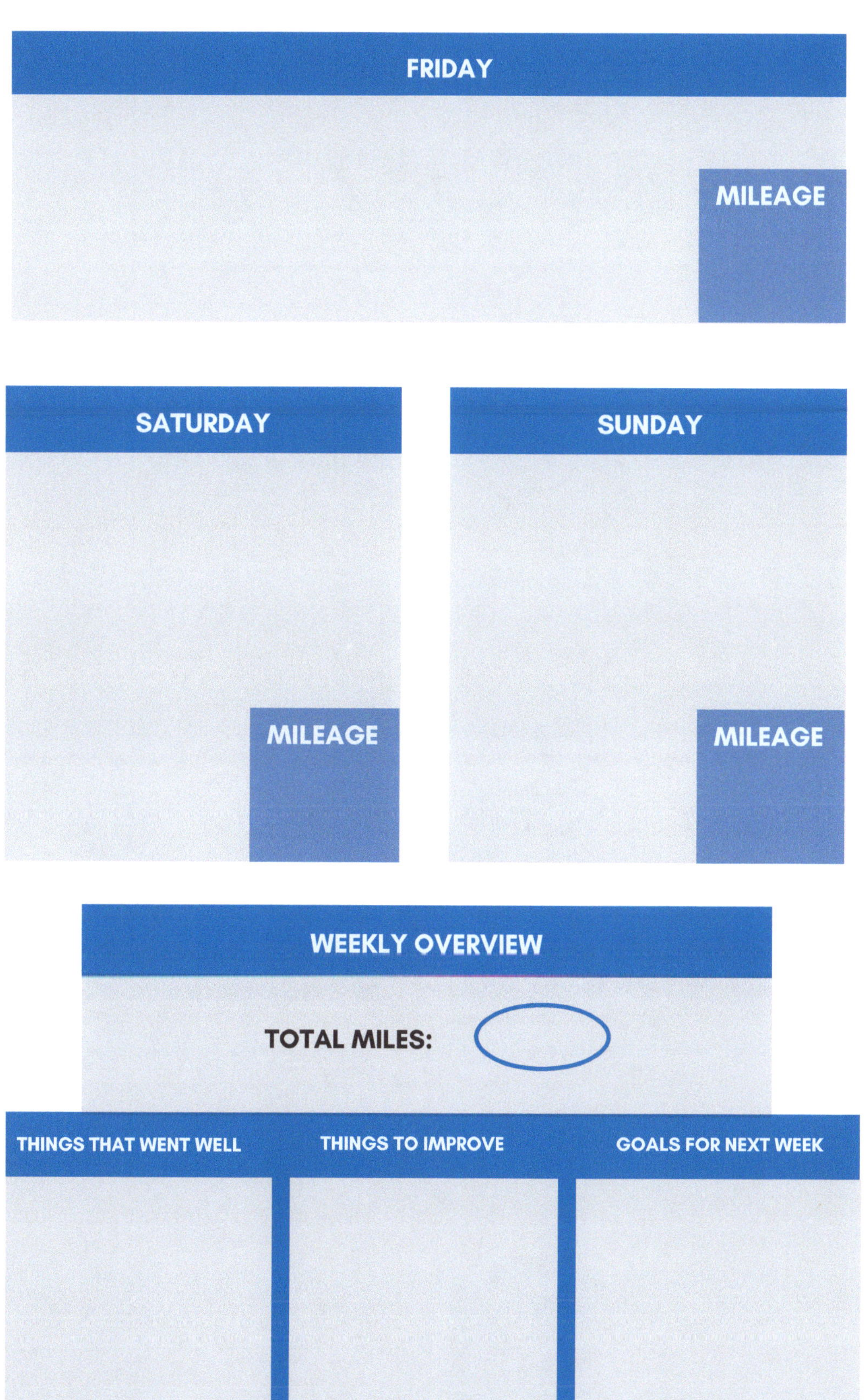

FRIDAY
MILEAGE
SATURDAY
MILEAGE
SUNDAY
MILEAGE
WEEKLY OVERVIEW
TOTAL MILES:
THINGS THAT WENT WELL
THINGS TO IMPROVE
GOALS FOR NEXT WEEK

WEEK OF:

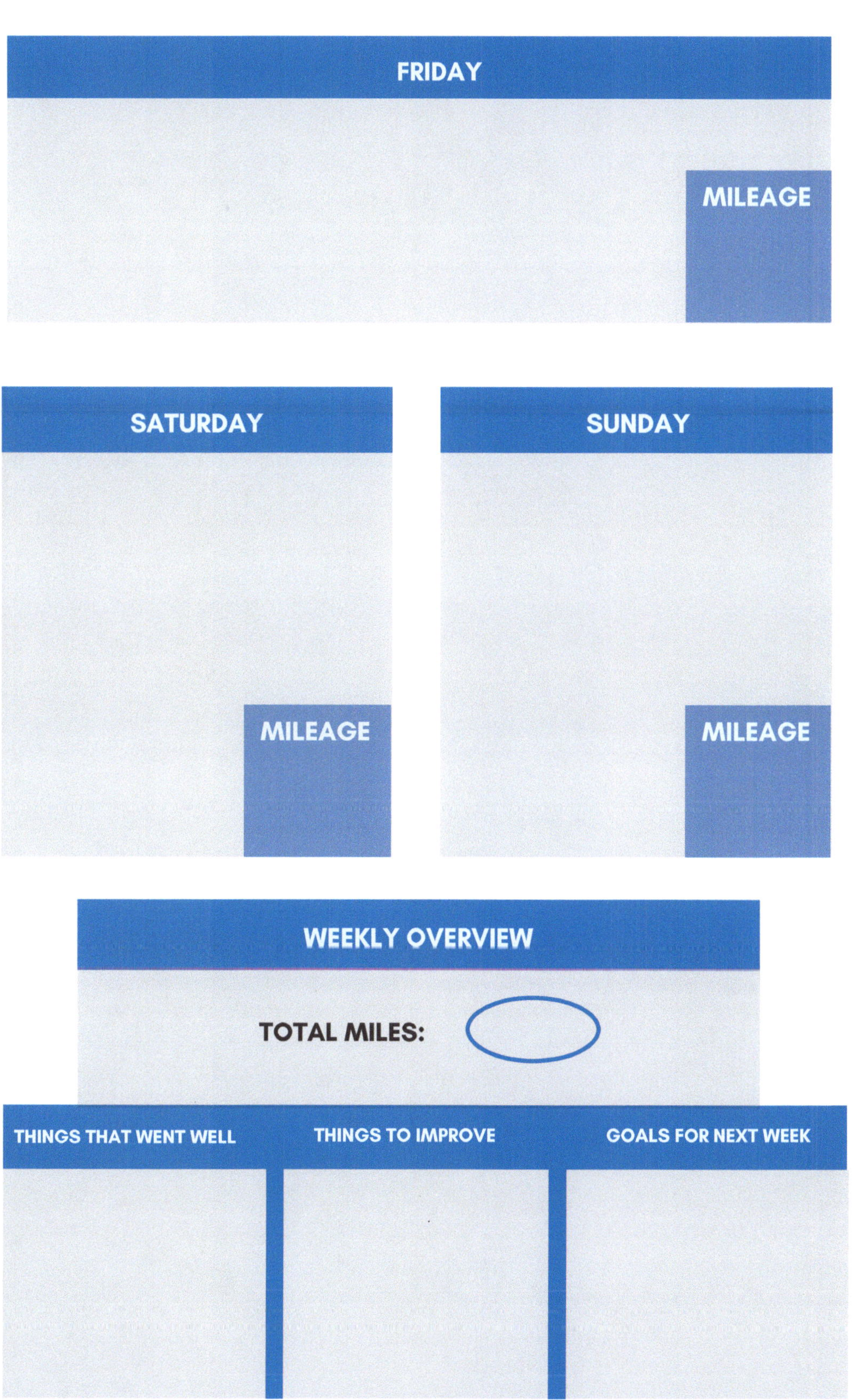

FRIDAY
MILEAGE
SATURDAY
MILEAGE
SUNDAY
MILEAGE
WEEKLY OVERVIEW
TOTAL MILES:
THINGS THAT WENT WELL
THINGS TO IMPROVE
GOALS FOR NEXT WEEK

WEEK OF:

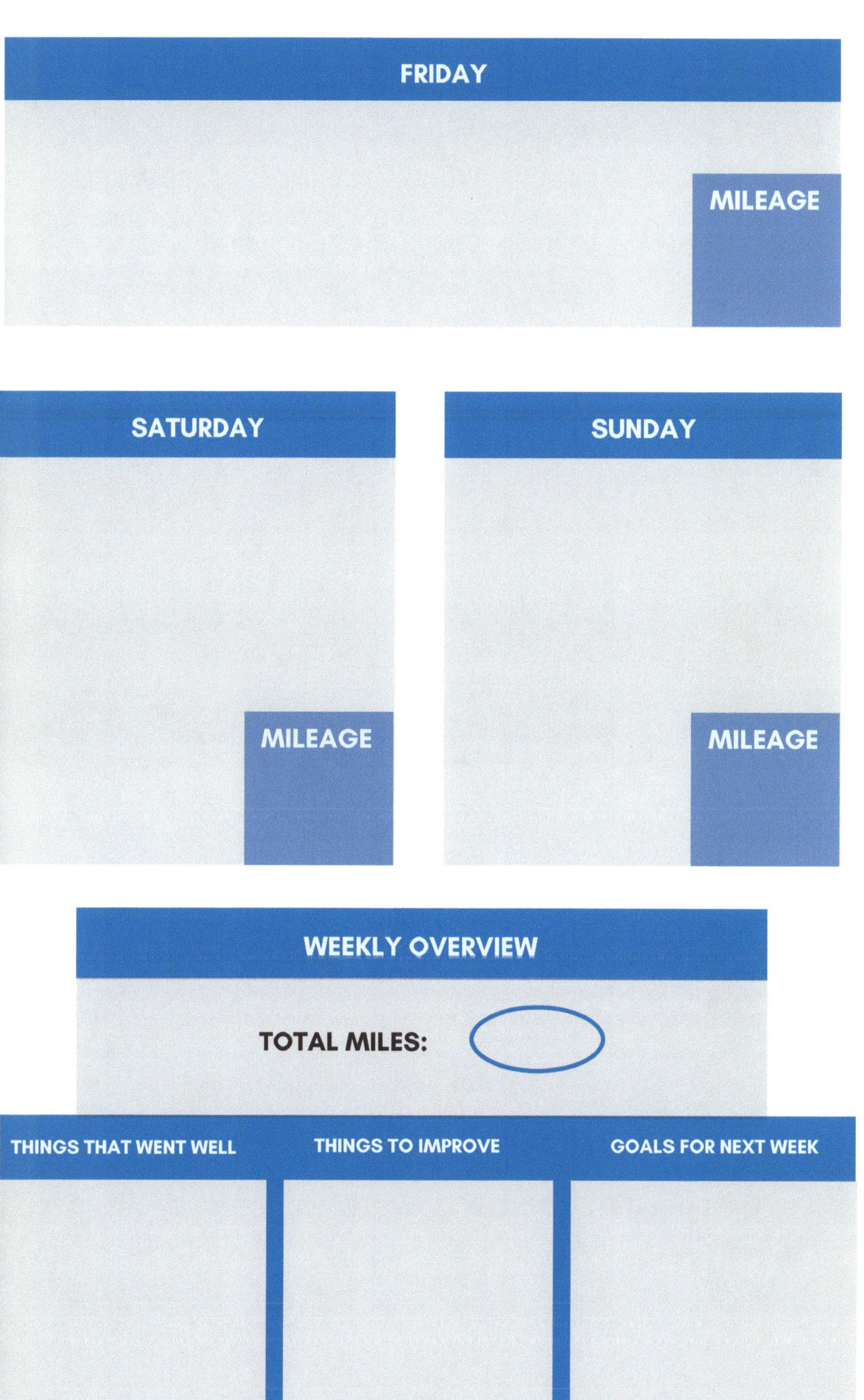

FRIDAY
MILEAGE
SATURDAY
MILEAGE
SUNDAY
MILEAGE
WEEKLY OVERVIEW
TOTAL MILES:
THINGS THAT WENT WELL
THINGS TO IMPROVE
GOALS FOR NEXT WEEK

RACE NAME	DATE	TIME	PLACE	HOW I FELT

YEARLY MILEAGE

JANUARY

FEBRUARY

MARCH

APRIL

MAY

JUNE

JULY

AUGUST

SEPTEMBER

OCTOBER

NOVEMBER

DECEMBER

TOTAL